Gastric Sleeve
Bariatric
Cookbook

Jerry V. Hatcher

i

Table of Contents

Introduction

Dear Readers,

Welcome to the "Gastric Sleeve Bariatric Cookbook" — a labor of love crafted with the well-being of your post-surgery journey in mind. In these pages, you'll discover a collection of recipes designed to nourish not only your body but also your spirit as you navigate the path to a healthier, more vibrant life.

Embarking on the journey of gastric sleeve surgery is a courageous step towards transformation, and it's our sincere hope that this cookbook becomes a trusted companion on your road to recovery. We understand the unique challenges and triumphs that accompany such a profound change in lifestyle, and it is with great empathy and enthusiasm that we present these recipes tailored specifically for your needs.

As you explore the chapters within, you'll find a variety of dishes that celebrate flavor, nutrition, and the joy of savoring each moment. From protein-packed breakfasts to wholesome lunches, satisfying dinners, and indulgent desserts (in moderation), each recipe is thoughtfully crafted to align with the dietary guidelines post-gastric sleeve surgery.

However, this cookbook extends beyond being a mere assortment of recipes; it's a celebration of your strength, resilience, and commitment to a healthier you. Within these pages, we share not only culinary creations but also practical tips, heartfelt stories, and a supportive community. This is a space where food becomes a source of nourishment, comfort, and joy.

As you commence this gastronomic journey, keep in mind that you have companions on the way. Whether you're seeking inspiration for a weeknight dinner or a special celebration, we're here to guide you with recipes that are not only delicious but also mindful of your unique nutritional needs.

May this cookbook be a source of inspiration, encouragement, and delight on your journey to wellness. Here's to savoring the flavors of a new chapter and embracing the nourishment that extends beyond the plate.

Wishing you health, happiness, and a table filled with love,

Jerry V. Hatcher

Author, Gastric Sleeve Bariatric Cookbook

About Gastric Sleeve Surgery

Gastric Sleeve Surgery, also known as sleeve gastrectomy, is a bariatric surgical procedure designed to assist individuals in achieving weight loss and improving overall health. This surgical intervention involves the removal of a large portion of the stomach, leaving behind a smaller, sleeve-shaped stomach resembling a banana or sleeve, hence the name.

The Procedure:

During the surgery, the surgeon removes approximately 75-85% of the stomach, reducing its capacity significantly. This reduction in stomach size leads to a decrease in the production of the hunger hormone, ghrelin, helping patients feel full with smaller portions of food. Unlike some other bariatric procedures, gastric sleeve surgery does not involve rerouting the intestines.

Benefits:

1. Effective Weight Loss: Gastric sleeve surgery is often successful in helping individuals achieve significant and sustained weight loss.

2. Improvement in Health Conditions: Many individuals experience improvements or remission in obesity-related health conditions such as type 2 diabetes, hypertension, and sleep apnea.

3. Enhanced Quality of Life: Weight loss following gastric sleeve surgery can lead to increased mobility, improved self-esteem, and a better overall quality of life.

Considerations:

1. Permanent Procedure: Gastric sleeve surgery is irreversible. Once the stomach is removed, it cannot be reattached.

2. Lifestyle Changes: Post-surgery, individuals are required to make substantial lifestyle changes, including adopting a nutritious and balanced diet, regular exercise, and ongoing medical monitoring.

3. Consultation and Eligibility: Candidates for gastric sleeve surgery undergo a thorough evaluation by healthcare professionals to determine their eligibility. This assessment includes considerations of the patient's overall health, BMI (Body Mass Index), and their commitment to the necessary lifestyle changes.

Post-Surgery:

After the surgery, patients typically follow a gradual dietary progression, starting with clear liquids and advancing to solid foods over several weeks. Regular follow-up appointments with healthcare providers, including dietitians, are essential to monitor progress and address any challenges.

Emotional and Psychological Support:

The journey through gastric sleeve surgery involves not only physical changes but also emotional and psychological adjustments. Many individuals find support through counseling, support groups, and a strong network of friends and family.

It's important to note that while gastric sleeve surgery can be a powerful tool for weight loss, its success is often closely tied to the individual's commitment to making sustainable lifestyle changes. As with any medical procedure, it's crucial for individuals to consult with healthcare professionals to determine the most suitable approach for their unique circumstances.

Nutritional Needs Post-Surgery

Gastric sleeve surgery marks the beginning of a transformative journey toward improved health and well-being. As you embark on this path, understanding and meeting your nutritional needs are essential for a successful recovery and long-term success. Here's a guide to help you navigate the post-surgery nutritional landscape:

1. Protein is Paramount:

   - Prioritize protein-rich foods to support healing, muscle maintenance, and satiety.

   - Include lean meats, poultry, fish, eggs, dairy, legumes, and plant-based protein sources in your meals.

2. Hydration is Crucial:

   - Sip water throughout the day to stay hydrated.

   - Limit caffeinated and carbonated beverages, as they may contribute to dehydration.

3. Micronutrient Mastery:

 - Consume a variety of colorful fruits and vegetables to obtain essential vitamins and minerals.

 - Consider vitamin and mineral supplements, as advised by your healthcare provider, to prevent deficiencies.

4. Mindful Carbohydrates:

 - Choose complex carbohydrates like whole grains, fruits, and vegetables over refined sugars.

 - Be mindful of portion sizes to avoid overconsumption.

5. Healthy Fats for Satiety:

 - Incorporate sources of healthy fats such as avocados, nuts, seeds, and olive oil.

 - Monitor portion sizes to manage calorie intake.

6. Structured Meal Plans:

 - Adopt a routine of small, frequent meals to prevent overeating and promote digestion.

- Listen to your body's hunger and fullness cues.

7. Limit Processed Foods:

- Minimize intake of processed and high-calorie, low-nutrient foods.

- Choose nutrient-dense options to maximize nutritional benefits.

8. Slow and Steady Introductions:

- Gradually reintroduce solid foods based on your healthcare provider's guidance.

- Monitor how your body responds to different foods and adjust your diet accordingly.

9. Regular Monitoring:

- Attend follow-up appointments with your healthcare team to assess nutritional status and address any concerns.

- Keep a food journal to track your intake and identify patterns.

10. Embrace Support and Education:

 - Join support groups or seek the guidance of a registered dietitian to navigate nutritional challenges.

 - Stay informed about your dietary requirements and make informed choices.

11. Physical Activity as a Complement:

 - Engage in regular physical activity suitable for your fitness level and post-surgery restrictions.

 - Exercise contributes to overall well-being and aids in weight management.

12. Listen to Your Body:

 - Pay attention to how your body responds to different foods.

 - Adjust your diet based on individual tolerances and preferences.

Your nutritional needs will evolve throughout your post-surgery journey. Regular communication with your healthcare team, along with a commitment to making informed dietary choices, will contribute to a successful and fulfilling recovery. Embrace the opportunity to nourish your body, mind, and spirit on this transformative path to a healthier you.

Foods to Avoid

After gastric sleeve surgery, it's crucial to be mindful of the foods you consume to support proper healing, prevent complications, and maximize the benefits of the surgery. Here are some general guidelines on foods to avoid:

1. High-Calorie, Low-Nutrient Foods:

   - Steer clear of foods that are high in calories but low in nutritional value, such as sugary snacks, candies, and sodas.

2. Highly Processed Foods:

   - Minimize the intake of heavily processed and refined foods, as they often lack essential nutrients and may contribute to weight gain.

3. Fried and Greasy Foods:

 - Avoid fried and greasy foods, as they can be difficult to digest and may cause discomfort.

4. Carbonated Beverages:

 - Limit or avoid carbonated beverages, as they can cause gas and bloating. Additionally, the carbonation may stretch the stomach.

5. Tough and Fibrous Meats:

 - Choose lean, tender meats and avoid tough or fibrous cuts that can be challenging to digest.

6. Large Portions:

 - Be cautious with portion sizes to prevent overeating. Consuming large portions can lead to discomfort and may interfere with weight loss goals.

7. Alcohol:

 - Limit or avoid alcohol as it can have a more pronounced effect post-surgery. It's essential to consult with your healthcare provider regarding alcohol consumption.

8. Sugary and High-Fat Foods:

   - Be mindful of sugary and high-fat foods, such as pastries, cakes, and fried snacks. These can contribute to excessive calorie intake.

9. Tough Raw Vegetables:

   - Choose cooked vegetables over raw ones, especially in the early stages of recovery. Raw, fibrous vegetables may be harder to digest.

10. Large Amounts of Dairy:

   - Gradually introduce dairy products and monitor for tolerance. Some individuals may experience lactose intolerance after surgery.

11. Bread and Dense Carbohydrates:

   - Opt for whole grains in moderation and avoid dense, doughy bread products that may cause discomfort.

12. Sugary Beverages and Juices:

   - Limit the intake of sugary beverages and fruit juices, as they contribute to unnecessary calorie intake without providing significant nutritional benefits.

13. Snacking Throughout the Day:

   - Instead of frequent snacking, focus on structured meals. Grazing throughout the day may hinder weight loss efforts.

It's crucial to note that individual tolerances may vary, and these guidelines are general recommendations. Consult with your healthcare team, including a registered dietitian, to tailor dietary advice to your specific needs and stage of recovery. Pay attention to your body's signals, and make adjustments to your diet based on your individual experiences and recommendations from your healthcare providers.

Chapter 1: Breakfast Delights

1. Protein-Packed Smoothie Bowl

Blend together a mix of low-fat Greek yogurt, a handful of berries, a scoop of protein powder, and a splash of almond milk. Top with sliced almonds and chia seeds for added texture and nutritional value.

Ingredients:

- 1/2 cup low-fat Greek yogurt

- 1/2 cup mixed berries (strawberries, blueberries, raspberries)

- 1 scoop protein powder

- 1/2 cup unsweetened almond milk

- 1 tablespoon sliced almonds

- 1 tablespoon chia seeds

Instructions:

1. Blend Greek yogurt, mixed berries, protein powder, and almond milk until smooth.

2. Pour the smoothie into a bowl.

3. Top with sliced almonds and chia seeds.

4. Enjoy with a spoon!

Nutritional Information (approximate):

- Calories: 250

- Protein: 25g

- Carbohydrates: 20g

- Fat: 8g

- Fiber: 5g

2. Veggie and Egg Breakfast Muffins

Whisk together eggs and fold in diced vegetables such as bell peppers, spinach, and tomatoes. Pour the mixture into muffin tins and bake until set. These portable muffins provide a protein-packed start to your day.

Ingredients:

- 4 large eggs

- 1/2 cup diced bell peppers

- 1/2 cup chopped spinach

- Salt and pepper to taste

Instructions:

1. Preheat the oven to 350°F (175°C).

2. In a bowl, whisk eggs and mix in diced bell peppers and chopped spinach.

3. Pour the mixture into greased muffin tins.

4. Bake for 15-20 minutes or until the eggs are set.

5. Allow to cool slightly before serving.

Nutritional Information (approximate):

- Calories: 150

- Protein: 12g

- Carbohydrates: 3g

- Fat: 10g

- Fiber: 1g

3. Greek Yogurt Parfait with Berries

Layer non-fat Greek yogurt with fresh berries and a sprinkle of granola. This parfait is not only delicious but also rich in protein and antioxidants.

Ingredients:

- 1 cup non-fat Greek yogurt

- 1/2 cup mixed berries (strawberries, blueberries, raspberries)

- 2 tablespoons granola

Instructions:

1. In a glass or bowl, layer Greek yogurt with mixed berries.

2. Top with granola just before serving.

Nutritional Information (approximate):

- Calories: 250

- Protein: 20g

- Carbohydrates: 35g

- Fat: 4g

- Fiber: 5g

4. Quinoa Breakfast Bowl

Cook quinoa and top it with sliced bananas, a drizzle of honey, and a sprinkle of cinnamon. Quinoa adds a protein boost to this nutrient-packed breakfast.

Ingredients:

- 1/2 cup cooked quinoa

- 1 medium banana, sliced

- 1 tablespoon honey

- 1/4 teaspoon cinnamon

Instructions:

1. In a bowl, combine cooked quinoa with sliced banana.

2. Drizzle with honey and sprinkle with cinnamon.

3. Stir gently and enjoy.

Nutritional Information (approximate):

- Calories: 300

- Protein: 7g

- Carbohydrates: 65g

- Fat: 2g

- Fiber: 6g

5. Spinach and Feta Egg Wrap

Fill a whole-grain tortilla with scrambled eggs, sautéed spinach, and crumbled feta cheese. This savory wrap is a satisfying way to start your day.

Ingredients:

- 2 large eggs, scrambled

- 1 cup fresh spinach, sautéed

- 2 tablespoons crumbled feta cheese

- 1 whole-grain tortilla

Instructions:

1. Scramble the eggs and set aside.

2. Sauté fresh spinach until wilted.

3. Warm the tortilla and fill with scrambled eggs, sautéed spinach, and crumbled feta.

4. Roll into a wrap and enjoy.

Nutritional Information (approximate):

- Calories: 300

- Protein: 20g

- Carbohydrates: 20g

- Fat: 15g

- Fiber: 5g

6. Almond Butter and Banana Rice Cakes

Spread almond butter on brown rice cakes and top with banana slices. This quick and easy breakfast provides a good balance of protein and healthy fats.

Ingredients:

- 2 brown rice cakes

- 2 tablespoons almond butter

- 1 medium banana, sliced

Instructions:

1. Spread almond butter evenly on the rice cakes.

2. Top with banana slices.

3. Enjoy this simple and satisfying breakfast.

Nutritional Information (approximate):

- Calories: 300

- Protein: 8g

- Carbohydrates: 40g

- Fat: 15g

- Fiber: 6g

7. Cottage Cheese and Pineapple Parfait

Layer low-fat cottage cheese with fresh pineapple chunks and a sprinkle of shredded coconut. This parfait is a tropical-inspired, protein-rich delight.

Ingredients:

- 1 cup low-fat cottage cheese

- 1/2 cup fresh pineapple chunks

- 1 tablespoon shredded coconut

Instructions:

1. In a glass or bowl, layer cottage cheese with fresh pineapple chunks.

2. Top with shredded coconut just before serving.

Nutritional Information (approximate):

- Calories: 250

- Protein: 25g

- Carbohydrates: 20g

- Fat: 8g

- Fiber: 2g

8. Baked Egg Avocado Boats

Hollow out an avocado half, crack an egg into the center, and bake until the egg is cooked to your liking. Sprinkle with herbs for added flavor.

Ingredients:

- 1 avocado, halved and pitted

- 2 eggs

- Salt and pepper to taste

- Fresh herbs for garnish (optional)

Instructions:

1. Preheat the oven to 375°F (190°C).

2. Scoop out a small portion of the avocado to create space for the egg.

3. Crack one egg into each avocado half.

4. Season with salt and pepper.

5. Bake for 12-15 minutes or until the eggs are cooked to your liking.

6. Garnish with fresh herbs if desired.

Nutritional Information (approximate):

- Calories: 300

- Protein: 12g

- Carbohydrates: 15g

- Fat: 24g

- Fiber: 10g

9. Chia Seed Pudding with Berries

Mix chia seeds with almond milk and let it sit overnight. Top with fresh berries in the morning for a fiber-rich and protein-packed pudding.

Ingredients:

- 2 tablespoons chia seeds

- 1/2 cup unsweetened almond milk

- 1/2 cup mixed berries (strawberries, blueberries, raspberries)

Instructions:

1. Mix chia seeds with almond milk in a jar or bowl.

2. Refrigerate overnight or for at least 2 hours until the mixture thickens.

3. Top with mixed berries before serving.

Nutritional Information (approximate):

- Calories: 200

- Protein: 5g

- Carbohydrates: 25g

- Fat: 10g

- Fiber: 10g

10. Breakfast Burrito Bowl

Create a burrito bowl with scrambled eggs, black beans, diced tomatoes, and a sprinkle of cheese. Customize with salsa and avocado for added flavor.

Ingredients:

- 2 scrambled eggs

- 1/2 cup black beans, drained and rinsed

- 1/2 cup diced tomatoes

- 2 tablespoons shredded cheese

- Salsa and sliced avocado for garnish

Instructions:

1. Scramble the eggs and set aside.

2. In a bowl, layer black beans, diced tomatoes, and scrambled eggs.

3. Top with shredded cheese, salsa, and sliced avocado.

Nutritional Information (approximate):

- Calories: 350

- Protein: 20g

- Carbohydrates: 25g

- Fat: 18g

- Fiber: 8g

Chapter 2: Wholesome Lunches

1. Grilled Chicken and Avocado Salad

Grilled chicken breast slices atop a bed of mixed greens, cherry tomatoes, cucumber, and avocado. Drizzle with a light vinaigrette for a refreshing and protein-packed salad.

Ingredients:

- 4 oz grilled chicken breast, sliced

- 2 cups mixed greens

- 1/2 cup cherry tomatoes, halved

- 1/2 cucumber, sliced

- 1/2 avocado, diced

- Light vinaigrette dressing

Instructions:

1. Arrange mixed greens on a plate.

2. Top with grilled chicken, cherry tomatoes, cucumber, and diced avocado.

3. Drizzle with light vinaigrette dressing.

Nutritional Information (approximate):

- Calories: 350

- Protein: 30g

- Carbohydrates: 15g

- Fat: 18g

- Fiber: 8g

2. Quinoa and Roasted Vegetable Stuffed Peppers

Colorful bell peppers stuffed with a mix of cooked quinoa, roasted zucchini, cherry tomatoes, and feta cheese. Baked until tender, these stuffed peppers offer a satisfying and nutrient-rich meal.

Ingredients:

- 2 large bell peppers, halved

- 1 cup cooked quinoa

- 1 cup roasted zucchini, cherry tomatoes, and feta cheese (mixed)

- Olive oil, salt, and pepper

Instructions:

1. Preheat the oven to 375°F (190°C).

2. Place bell pepper halves on a baking sheet.

3. Fill each half with a mix of cooked quinoa, roasted vegetables, and feta cheese.

4. Drizzle with olive oil and season with salt and pepper.

5. Bake for 25-30 minutes or until peppers are tender.

Nutritional Information (approximate):

- Calories: 300

- Protein: 12g

- Carbohydrates: 40g

- Fat: 10g

- Fiber: 8g

3. Spinach and Feta Turkey Burgers

Lean ground turkey blended with spinach, feta cheese, and Mediterranean spices. Grill or bake the patties and serve with whole-grain buns or lettuce wraps for a flavorful burger alternative.

Ingredients:

- 1 lb lean ground turkey

- 1 cup chopped spinach

- 1/2 cup crumbled feta cheese

- 1 tsp dried oregano

- Salt and pepper to taste

- Whole-grain buns or lettuce wraps

Instructions:

1. In a bowl, mix ground turkey, chopped spinach, feta cheese, oregano, salt, and pepper.

2. Form into burger patties.

3. Grill or bake until cooked through.

4. Serve on whole-grain buns or lettuce wraps.

Nutritional Information (approximate):

- Calories: 250

- Protein: 30g

- Carbohydrates: 5g

- Fat: 12g

- Fiber: 2g

4. Baked Salmon with Lemon-Dill Sauce

Oven-baked salmon fillet seasoned with lemon and dill. Serve alongside steamed asparagus and quinoa for a heart-healthy and protein-rich lunch.

Ingredients:

- 6 oz salmon fillet

- 1 tbsp olive oil

- Lemon slices

- Fresh dill, chopped

- Salt and pepper to taste

- Steamed asparagus

- 1/2 cup cooked quinoa

Instructions:

1. Preheat the oven to 400°F (200°C).

2. Place salmon on a baking sheet.

3. Drizzle with olive oil, season with salt and pepper, and top with lemon slices and chopped dill.

4. Bake for 15-20 minutes or until salmon flakes easily.

5. Serve with steamed asparagus and quinoa.

Nutritional Information (approximate):

- Calories: 400

- Protein: 30g

- Carbohydrates: 20g

- Fat: 20g

- Fiber: 3g

5. Zucchini Noodles with Pesto and Cherry Tomatoes

Spiralized zucchini noodles tossed with homemade basil pesto and cherry tomatoes. This low-carb alternative to traditional pasta is light, flavorful, and packed with nutrients.

Ingredients:

- 2 medium zucchinis, spiralized

- 2 tbsp homemade or store-bought basil pesto

- 1 cup cherry tomatoes, halved

- Parmesan cheese (optional)

Instructions:

1. Spiralize zucchinis to create noodles.

2. Toss zucchini noodles with basil pesto.

3. Top with cherry tomatoes and Parmesan cheese if desired.

Nutritional Information (approximate):

- Calories: 200

- Protein: 5g

- Carbohydrates: 15g

- Fat: 15g

- Fiber: 5g

6. Lean Beef Stir-Fry with Broccoli and Ginger

Thinly sliced lean beef stir-fried with colorful vegetables like broccoli, bell peppers, and snap peas. Seasoned with ginger and garlic for a delicious and protein-packed stir-fry.

Ingredients:

- 4 oz lean beef strips

- 1 cup broccoli florets

- 1/2 bell pepper, sliced

- 1 cup snap peas

- 1 tbsp low-sodium soy sauce

- 1 tsp grated ginger

- 1 clove garlic, minced

- 1 tsp sesame oil (optional)

- Brown rice (optional, for serving)

Instructions:

1. In a wok or skillet, stir-fry beef until browned.

2. Add broccoli, bell pepper, and snap peas.

3. Mix in soy sauce, ginger, and garlic.

4. Cook until vegetables are tender-crisp.

5. Drizzle with sesame oil if desired.

6. Serve alone or over brown rice.

Nutritional Information (approximate):

- Calories: 350

- Protein: 25g

- Carbohydrates: 20g

- Fat: 15g

- Fiber: 6g

7. Almond Butter and Turkey Lettuce Wraps

Sliced turkey breast spread with almond butter and wrapped in crisp lettuce leaves. Add thinly sliced apples or cucumbers for a satisfying and crunchy texture.

Ingredients:

- 4 oz sliced turkey breast

- 2 tbsp almond butter

- 4 large lettuce leaves

- 1/2 apple or cucumber, thinly sliced

Instructions:

1. Spread almond butter on each lettuce leaf.

2. Add turkey slices and apple or cucumber slices.

3. Wrap and secure with toothpicks if needed.

Nutritional Information (approximate):

- Calories: 300

- Protein: 20g

- Carbohydrates: 15g

- Fat: 15g

- Fiber: 5g

8. Quinoa Salad with Chickpeas and Mediterranean Veggies

A hearty salad featuring cooked quinoa, chickpeas, cherry tomatoes, cucumber, Kalamata olives, and feta cheese. Tossed in a lemon-oregano vinaigrette for a Mediterranean-inspired delight.

Ingredients:

- 1 cup cooked quinoa

- 1/2 cup canned chickpeas, drained and rinsed

- 1/2 cup cherry tomatoes, halved

- 1/4 cup Kalamata olives, sliced

- 1/4 cup feta cheese, crumbled

- Lemon-oregano vinaigrette

Instructions:

1. In a bowl, combine cooked quinoa, chickpeas, cherry tomatoes, olives, and feta.

2. Toss with lemon-oregano vinaigrette.

Nutritional Information (approximate):

- Calories: 350

- Protein: 12g

- Carbohydrates: 40g

- Fat: 15g

- Fiber: 8g

9. Turkey and Avocado Wrap with Whole-Grain Tortilla

Sliced turkey breast, avocado, lettuce, and tomato wrapped in a whole-grain tortilla. A convenient and balanced lunch option with a mix of protein, healthy fats, and fiber.

Ingredients:

- 4 oz sliced turkey breast

- 1/2 avocado, sliced

- 1 cup mixed greens

- 1 medium tomato, sliced

- Whole-grain tortilla

Instructions:

1. Lay out the tortilla and layer with turkey, avocado, mixed greens, and tomato.

2. Roll into a wrap and slice in half.

Nutritional Information (approximate):

- Calories: 300

- Protein: 20g

- Carbohydrates: 25g

- Fat: 15g

- Fiber: 8g

10. Chicken and Vegetable Skewers with Tzatziki

Skewers of grilled chicken breast, cherry tomatoes, bell peppers, and red onions served with a side of tzatziki sauce. A delicious and protein-rich option for a satisfying lunch.

Ingredients:

- 4 oz chicken breast, cut into cubes

- Cherry tomatoes

- Bell pepper, cut into chunks

- Red onion, cut into wedges

- Tzatziki sauce for dipping

Instructions:

1. Thread chicken, cherry tomatoes, bell pepper, and red onion onto skewers.

2. Grill or bake until chicken is cooked through.

3. Serve with a side of tzatziki sauce.

Nutritional Information (approximate):

- Calories: 250

- Protein: 25g

- Carbohydrates: 15g

- Fat: 10g

- Fiber: 4g

Chapter 3: Satisfying Dinners

1. Baked Lemon Herb Chicken with Roasted Vegetables

Juicy chicken breasts marinated in a lemon-herb blend, baked to perfection, and served with a side of colorful roasted vegetables.

Ingredients:

- 4 oz chicken breast

- 1 tablespoon olive oil

- 1 tablespoon lemon juice

- 1 teaspoon dried herbs (such as rosemary, thyme, or oregano)

- Salt and pepper to taste

- Assorted vegetables (e.g., bell peppers, zucchini, cherry tomatoes)

Instructions:

1. Preheat the oven to 400°F (200°C).

2. In a bowl, mix olive oil, lemon juice, dried herbs, salt, and pepper.

3. Coat the chicken with the mixture and place it on a baking sheet.

4. Surround the chicken with assorted vegetables.

5. Bake for 20-25 minutes or until the chicken is cooked through.

Nutritional Information (approximate):

- Calories: 350

- Protein: 30g

- Carbohydrates: 15g

- Fat: 18g

- Fiber: 5g

2. Cauliflower Fried Rice with Shrimp

A low-carb twist on fried rice using cauliflower rice, mixed with shrimp, vegetables, and soy sauce for a flavorful and satisfying meal.

Ingredients:

- 4 oz shrimp, peeled and deveined

- 1 cup cauliflower rice

- 1/2 cup mixed vegetables (peas, carrots, corn)

- 1 egg, beaten

- 1 tablespoon soy sauce

- 1 teaspoon sesame oil

- Green onions for garnish

Instructions:

1. In a pan, sauté shrimp until cooked. Remove and set aside.

2. Add cauliflower rice and mixed vegetables to the pan.

3. Push the veggies to the side and pour the beaten egg into the pan. Scramble.

4. Combine the egg with the veggies, add cooked shrimp, soy sauce, and sesame oil.

5. Stir well, garnish with green onions, and serve.

Nutritional Information (approximate):

- Calories: 300

- Protein: 25g

- Carbohydrates: 15g

- Fat: 15g

- Fiber: 5g

3. Turkey and Vegetable Chili

A lean turkey and vegetable chili, simmered with tomatoes, beans, and spices, providing warmth and protein without excessive calories.

Ingredients:

- 4 oz lean ground turkey

- 1/2 cup black beans, drained and rinsed

- 1/2 cup diced tomatoes

- 1/4 cup diced bell peppers

- 1/4 cup diced onions

- 1 clove garlic, minced

- Chili powder, cumin, salt, and pepper to taste

Instructions:

1. In a pan, cook ground turkey until browned.

2. Add diced tomatoes, black beans, bell peppers, onions, and garlic.

3. Season with chili powder, cumin, salt, and pepper.

4. Simmer for 15-20 minutes, stirring occasionally.

Nutritional Information (approximate):

- Calories: 250

- Protein: 20g

- Carbohydrates: 20g

- Fat: 10g

- Fiber: 8g

4. Salmon and Quinoa Stuffed Bell Peppers

Bell peppers stuffed with a mixture of flaked salmon, cooked quinoa, spinach, and herbs, baked until tender for a nutrient-packed dinner.

Ingredients:

- 6 oz salmon fillet, cooked and flaked

- 1/2 cup cooked quinoa

- 1 cup fresh spinach, chopped

- 2 bell peppers, halved

- Lemon juice, salt, and pepper to taste

- Optional: Feta cheese for garnish

Instructions:

1. Preheat the oven to 375°F (190°C).

2. In a bowl, mix salmon, cooked quinoa, chopped spinach, lemon juice, salt, and pepper.

3. Stuff bell pepper halves with the mixture.

4. Bake for 20-25 minutes.

5. Garnish with feta cheese if desired.

Nutritional Information (approximate):

- Calories: 350

- Protein: 25g

- Carbohydrates: 20g

- Fat: 18g

- Fiber: 5g

5. Zoodle (Zucchini Noodle) Bolognese

Zucchini noodles topped with a hearty turkey or lean beef Bolognese sauce, offering a comforting and low-carb alternative to traditional pasta.

Ingredients:

- 4 oz lean ground turkey or beef

- 1 cup zucchini noodles (zoodles)

- 1/2 cup diced tomatoes

- 1/4 cup tomato sauce

- 1 clove garlic, minced

- Italian herbs, salt, and pepper to taste

- Grated Parmesan cheese for garnish

Instructions:

1. In a pan, brown ground turkey or beef.

2. Add diced tomatoes, tomato sauce, garlic, and seasonings.

3. Simmer for 10-15 minutes.

4. Spiralize zucchini to create noodles and cook briefly.

5. Serve Bolognese sauce over zoodles.

6. Garnish with grated Parmesan.

Nutritional Information (approximate):

- Calories: 300

- Protein: 20g

- Carbohydrates: 15g

- Fat: 15g

- Fiber: 5g

6. Vegetarian Stir-Fry with Tofu and Broccoli

Tofu and broccoli stir-fried with colorful vegetables in a savory sauce, served over cauliflower rice for a plant-based and protein-rich dinner.

Ingredients:

- 4 oz firm tofu, cubed

- 1 cup broccoli florets

- 1/2 bell pepper, sliced

- 1 cup snap peas

- 1 tablespoon low-sodium soy sauce

- 1 teaspoon sesame oil

- 1 clove garlic, minced

- 1 teaspoon grated ginger

- Cauliflower rice for serving

Instructions:

1. In a wok or skillet, sauté tofu until golden brown.

2. Add broccoli, bell pepper, and snap peas.

3. Mix in soy sauce, sesame oil, garlic, and ginger.

4. Cook until vegetables are tender.

5. Serve over cauliflower rice.

Nutritional Information (approximate):

- Calories: 300

- Protein: 20g

- Carbohydrates: 15g

- Fat: 15g

- Fiber: 6g

7. Grilled Cilantro Lime Chicken with Avocado Salsa

Grilled chicken breasts seasoned with cilantro and lime, topped with a refreshing avocado salsa, creating a flavorful and satisfying dish.

Ingredients:

- 4 oz chicken breast

- 1 tablespoon olive oil

- 1 tablespoon fresh cilantro, chopped

- 1 lime, juiced

- Salt and pepper to taste

- Avocado salsa (diced avocado, tomato, red onion, lime juice)

Instructions:

1. In a bowl, mix olive oil, cilantro, lime juice, salt, and pepper.

2. Coat the chicken with the mixture and grill until cooked through.

3. Top with avocado salsa before serving.

Nutritional Information (approximate):

- Calories: 350

- Protein: 30g

- Carbohydrates: 15g

- Fat: 18g

- Fiber: 6g

8. Eggplant Lasagna with Ground Turkey

Layers of thinly sliced eggplant, lean ground turkey, marinara sauce, and ricotta cheese, baked to perfection for a low-carb twist on classic lasagna.

Ingredients:

- 4 oz lean ground turkey

- 1 medium eggplant, thinly sliced

- 1 cup marinara sauce (low-sugar)

- 1 cup part-skim ricotta cheese

- 1 cup shredded mozzarella cheese

- Italian herbs, salt, and pepper to taste

Instructions:

1. Preheat the oven to 375°F (190°C).

2. In a pan, cook ground turkey until browned. Season with herbs, salt, and pepper.

3. In a baking dish, layer sliced eggplant, turkey, marinara sauce, ricotta, and mozzarella.

4. Repeat layers and bake for 30-40 minutes.

Nutritional Information (approximate):

- Calories: 350

- Protein: 30g

- Carbohydrates: 20g

- Fat: 18g

- Fiber: 8g

9. Quinoa and Black Bean Stuffed Peppers

Bell peppers filled with a mixture of quinoa, black beans, corn, and spices, baked until tender, providing a protein-packed and satisfying meal.

Ingredients:

- 1/2 cup cooked quinoa

- 1/2 cup black beans, drained and rinsed

- 1/4 cup corn kernels

- 1/4 cup diced tomatoes

- 1/4 cup diced red onion

- 2 bell peppers, halved

- Mexican seasoning, salt, and pepper to taste

Instructions:

1. Preheat the oven to 375°F (190°C).

2. In a bowl, mix quinoa, black beans, corn, tomatoes, red onion, and seasonings.

3. Stuff bell pepper halves with the mixture.

4. Bake for 20-25 minutes.

Nutritional Information (approximate):

- Calories: 300

- Protein: 15g

- Carbohydrates: 50g

- Fat: 5g

- Fiber: 12g

10. Cajun Shrimp and Vegetable Skewers

Skewers of Cajun-seasoned shrimp, bell peppers, and cherry tomatoes, grilled to perfection and served with a side of quinoa or cauliflower rice.

Ingredients:

- 4 oz shrimp, peeled and deveined

- Cherry tomatoes

- Bell pepper, cut into chunks

- Red onion, cut into wedges

- Cajun seasoning, salt, and pepper to taste

- Quinoa or cauliflower rice for serving

Instructions:

1. Preheat the grill.

2. Thread shrimp, cherry tomatoes, bell pepper, and red onion onto skewers.

3. Season with Cajun seasoning, salt, and pepper.

4. Grill until shrimp are opaque.

5. Serve over quinoa or cauliflower rice.

Nutritional Information (approximate):

- Calories: 250

- Protein: 25g

- Carbohydrates: 15g

- Fat: 10g

- Fiber: 4g

Chapter 4: Nourishing Snacks

1. Greek Yogurt Parfait with Berries

A delightful snack featuring non-fat Greek yogurt layered with fresh berries and a sprinkle of granola for added crunch and fiber.

Ingredients:

- 1/2 cup non-fat Greek yogurt

- 1/4 cup mixed berries (strawberries, blueberries, raspberries)

- 2 tablespoons granola

Instructions:

1. In a glass or bowl, layer Greek yogurt with mixed berries.

2. Sprinkle granola on top.

3. Enjoy this delicious and protein-packed parfait.

Nutritional Information (approximate):

- Calories: 200

- Protein: 15g

- Carbohydrates: 30g

- Fat: 3g

- Fiber: 5g

2. Hard-Boiled Egg and Cherry Tomatoes

A protein-packed snack comprising hard-boiled eggs paired with sweet cherry tomatoes, providing a balance of nutrients and satiety.

Ingredients:

- 2 hard-boiled eggs

- 1/2 cup cherry tomatoes

- Salt and pepper to taste

Instructions:

1. Peel and slice hard-boiled eggs.

2. Serve with cherry tomatoes.

3. Season with salt and pepper.

Nutritional Information (approximate):

- Calories: 160

- Protein: 14g

- Carbohydrates: 4g

- Fat: 10g

- Fiber: 2g

3. Hummus and Veggie Sticks

Nutrient-rich hummus served alongside colorful vegetable sticks such as cucumber, bell peppers, and cherry tomatoes for a satisfying and flavorful snack.

Ingredients:

- 1/2 cup hummus

- Assorted vegetable sticks (cucumber, bell peppers, cherry tomatoes)

Instructions:

1. Arrange vegetable sticks on a plate.

2. Dip in hummus and enjoy this crunchy and satisfying snack.

Nutritional Information (approximate):

- Calories: 180

- Protein: 6g

- Carbohydrates: 20g

- Fat: 9g

- Fiber: 7g

4. Cottage Cheese and Pineapple Bowl

A simple yet tasty snack featuring low-fat cottage cheese paired with fresh pineapple chunks, offering a blend of protein and natural sweetness.

Ingredients:

- 1/2 cup low-fat cottage cheese

- 1/2 cup fresh pineapple chunks

Instructions:

1. In a bowl, combine cottage cheese with pineapple chunks.

2. Mix well and enjoy this simple and protein-rich snack.

Nutritional Information (approximate):

- Calories: 150

- Protein: 15g

- Carbohydrates: 20g

- Fat: 2g

- Fiber: 2g

5. Almond Butter and Apple Slices

Thin apple slices spread with almond butter, creating a satisfying combination of fiber, healthy fats, and a touch of sweetness.

Ingredients:

- 1 medium apple, sliced

- 2 tablespoons almond butter

Instructions:

1. Slice the apple into thin wedges.

2. Spread almond butter on each apple slice.

3. Enjoy this sweet and satisfying snack.

Nutritional Information (approximate):

- Calories: 200

- Protein: 4g

- Carbohydrates: 20g

- Fat: 12g

- Fiber: 5g

6. Protein-Packed Trail Mix

A custom trail mix blend featuring nuts, seeds, and a moderate amount of dried fruits for a portable and protein-rich snack.

Ingredients:

- 1/4 cup almonds

- 1/4 cup walnuts

- 2 tablespoons pumpkin seeds

- 2 tablespoons dried cranberries (unsweetened)

- 1 tablespoon dark chocolate chips

Instructions:

1. Mix all ingredients in a bowl.

2. Portion into snack-sized servings.

3. Enjoy this protein-rich and satisfying trail mix.

Nutritional Information (approximate):

- Calories: 250

- Protein: 7g

- Carbohydrates: 15g

- Fat: 18g

- Fiber: 4g

7. Chia Seed Pudding with Berries

Chia seeds soaked in almond milk and topped with mixed berries, creating a delicious and nutrient-dense pudding with a boost of omega-3 fatty acids.

Ingredients:

- 2 tablespoons chia seeds

- 1/2 cup almond milk

- 1/2 teaspoon vanilla extract

- Mixed berries for topping

Instructions:

1. Mix chia seeds, almond milk, and vanilla extract in a jar.

2. Refrigerate for at least 2 hours or overnight.

3. Top with mixed berries before serving.

Nutritional Information (approximate):

- Calories: 150

- Protein: 5g

- Carbohydrates: 20g

- Fat: 7g

- Fiber: 10g

8. Turkey and Cheese Roll-Ups

Deli turkey slices wrapped around light cheese sticks, offering a convenient and protein-rich snack with minimal carbohydrates.

Ingredients:

- 4 slices deli turkey

- 2 light cheese sticks

Instructions:

1. Lay out turkey slices.

2. Place a cheese stick on each slice.

3. Roll up and secure with toothpicks if needed.

Nutritional Information (approximate):

- Calories: 200

- Protein: 25g

- Carbohydrates: 2g

- Fat: 10g

- Fiber: 0g

9. Avocado and Tomato Salsa

Sliced avocado paired with a flavorful tomato salsa, served with whole-grain crackers for a satisfying blend of healthy fats and fiber.

Ingredients:

- 1/2 avocado, diced

- 1/2 cup diced tomatoes

- 1/4 cup red onion, finely chopped

- Fresh cilantro, chopped

- Whole-grain crackers for serving

Instructions:

1. In a bowl, mix avocado, tomatoes, red onion, and cilantro.

2. Serve with whole-grain crackers.

Nutritional Information (approximate):

- Calories: 180

- Protein: 2g

- Carbohydrates: 15g

- Fat: 12g

- Fiber: 6g

10. Roasted Chickpeas

Crunchy and savory roasted chickpeas seasoned with herbs and spices, providing a high-fiber and protein-packed alternative to traditional snacks.

Ingredients:

- 1 can (15 oz) chickpeas, drained and rinsed

- 1 tablespoon olive oil

- 1 teaspoon smoked paprika

- 1/2 teaspoon cumin

- Salt and pepper to taste

Instructions:

1. Preheat the oven to 400°F (200°C).

2. Toss chickpeas with olive oil, smoked paprika, cumin, salt, and pepper.

3. Spread on a baking sheet and roast for 25-30 minutes until crispy.

Nutritional Information (approximate):

- Calories: 200

- Protein: 7g

- Carbohydrates: 30g

- Fat: 6g

- Fiber: 7g

Chapter 5: Indulgent Desserts (In Moderation)

1. Dark Chocolate Avocado Mousse

A rich and creamy mousse made with ripe avocados, unsweetened cocoa powder, and a touch of honey, providing a decadent chocolate treat with healthy fats.

Ingredients:

- 1 ripe avocado

- 2 tablespoons unsweetened cocoa powder

- 2 tablespoons honey or maple syrup

- 1/2 teaspoon vanilla extract

- Pinch of salt

Instructions:

1. In a blender, combine avocado, cocoa powder, honey or maple syrup, vanilla extract, and a pinch of salt.

2. Blend until smooth and creamy.

3. Refrigerate for at least 30 minutes before serving.

Nutritional Information (approximate):

- Calories: 200

- Protein: 3g

- Carbohydrates: 20g

- Fat: 15g

- Fiber: 7g

2. Protein-Packed Peanut Butter Balls

Bite-sized balls made with a blend of protein powder, peanut butter, and a hint of honey, offering a satisfying and sweet treat that's high in protein.

Ingredients:

- 1/2 cup protein powder (whey or plant-based)

- 1/2 cup peanut butter

- 2 tablespoons honey

- 1/2 teaspoon vanilla extract

- Shredded coconut for coating (optional)

Instructions:

1. In a bowl, mix protein powder, peanut butter, honey, and vanilla extract until well combined.

2. Roll the mixture into small balls.

3. Optional: Roll the balls in shredded coconut.

4. Refrigerate for 1 hour before serving.

Nutritional Information (approximate):

- Calories: 150

- Protein: 8g

- Carbohydrates: 8g

- Fat: 10g

- Fiber: 2g

3. Baked Apple with Cinnamon and Almonds

An oven-baked apple sprinkled with cinnamon and topped with chopped almonds, providing a warm and comforting dessert without added sugars.

Ingredients:

- 1 apple, cored and sliced

- 1/2 teaspoon cinnamon

- 1 tablespoon chopped almonds

- 1 teaspoon honey (optional)

Instructions:

1. Preheat the oven to 375°F (190°C).

2. Place apple slices in a baking dish.

3. Sprinkle with cinnamon and chopped almonds.

4. Drizzle with honey if desired.

5. Bake for 20-25 minutes until apples are tender.

Nutritional Information (approximate):

- Calories: 120

- Protein: 2g

- Carbohydrates: 25g

- Fat: 3g

- Fiber: 5g

4. Greek Yogurt Berry Parfait

Layers of non-fat Greek yogurt, mixed berries, and a drizzle of honey or a sprinkle of granola, creating a parfait that's both indulgent and high in protein.

Ingredients:

- 1/2 cup non-fat Greek yogurt

- 1/4 cup mixed berries (strawberries, blueberries, raspberries)

- 1 tablespoon honey or a sprinkle of granola

Instructions:

1. In a glass or bowl, layer Greek yogurt with mixed berries.

2. Drizzle with honey or sprinkle with granola.

3. Enjoy this high-protein parfait.

Nutritional Information (approximate):

- Calories: 150

- Protein: 15g

- Carbohydrates: 20g

- Fat: 0g

- Fiber: 3g

5. Coconut Chia Seed Pudding

Creamy chia seed pudding made with coconut milk, topped with fresh berries or a small amount of shredded coconut, offering a tropical and satisfying dessert.

Ingredients:

- 2 tablespoons chia seeds

- 1/2 cup coconut milk

- 1/2 teaspoon vanilla extract

- Fresh berries or shredded coconut for topping

Instructions:

1. In a jar, mix chia seeds, coconut milk, and vanilla extract.

2. Refrigerate for at least 2 hours or overnight.

3. Top with fresh berries or shredded coconut before serving.

Nutritional Information (approximate):

- Calories: 180

- Protein: 4g

- Carbohydrates: 15g

- Fat: 12g

- Fiber: 8g

6. Almond Flour Banana Bread

Moist and flavorful banana bread made with almond flour, ripe bananas, and a touch of cinnamon, providing a gluten-free and higher protein alternative.

Ingredients:

- 2 ripe bananas, mashed

- 2 eggs

- 1 teaspoon vanilla extract

- 1 cup almond flour

- 1/2 teaspoon baking soda

- 1/4 teaspoon salt

- Optional: Cinnamon or nutmeg for flavor

Instructions:

1. Preheat the oven to 350°F (175°C) and grease a loaf pan.

2. In a bowl, mix mashed bananas, eggs, and vanilla extract.

3. Add almond flour, baking soda, salt, and optional spices. Mix well.

4. Pour the batter into the prepared pan and bake for 25-30 minutes or until a toothpick comes out clean.

Nutritional Information (approximate):

- Calories: 180

- Protein: 6g

- Carbohydrates: 15g

- Fat: 12g

- Fiber: 3g

7. Berry and Almond Crumble

A delightful crumble featuring mixed berries topped with a mixture of almond flour, oats, and a small amount of butter or coconut oil, creating a delicious and satisfying dessert.

Ingredients:

- 1 cup mixed berries (strawberries, blueberries, raspberries)

- 1/4 cup almond flour

- 1/4 cup oats

- 2 tablespoons butter or coconut oil, melted

- 1 tablespoon honey or maple syrup

- Pinch of salt

Instructions:

1. Preheat the oven to 350°F (175°C).

2. In a bowl, mix berries with almond flour, oats, melted butter or coconut oil, honey or maple syrup, and a pinch of salt.

3. Transfer the mixture to a baking dish and bake for 20-25 minutes or until the top is golden brown.

Nutritional Information (approximate):

- Calories: 200

- Protein: 3g

- Carbohydrates: 20g

- Fat: 12g

- Fiber: 5g

8. Vanilla Protein Ice Cream

Homemade ice cream made with protein powder, almond milk, and vanilla extract, offering a guilt-free and protein-packed alternative to traditional ice cream.

Ingredients:

- 2 cups unsweetened almond milk

- 1 scoop vanilla protein powder

- 1 teaspoon vanilla extract

- Optional: Stevia or sweetener of choice to taste

Instructions:

1. Blend almond milk, vanilla protein powder, vanilla extract, and sweetener until smooth.

2. Pour the mixture into an ice cream maker and churn according to the manufacturer's instructions.

3. Transfer to a container and freeze for an additional 2 hours before serving.

Nutritional Information (approximate):

- Calories: 120

- Protein: 15g

- Carbohydrates: 3g

- Fat: 6g

- Fiber: 1g

9. Cocoa-Dusted Almonds

Almonds dusted with unsweetened cocoa powder and a touch of stevia or powdered sugar, providing a crunchy and chocolatey snack in moderation.

Ingredients:

- 1 cup raw almonds

- 2 tablespoons unsweetened cocoa powder

- 1-2 tablespoons powdered sugar or stevia (optional)

Instructions:

1. In a bowl, toss raw almonds with cocoa powder until well coated.

2. Optional: Add powdered sugar or stevia for sweetness.

3. Spread the almonds on a baking sheet and let them dry completely.

Nutritional Information (approximate):

- Calories: 180

- Protein: 7g

- Carbohydrates: 10g

- Fat: 14g

- Fiber: 6g

10. Pumpkin Spice Protein Bites

Energy bites made with pumpkin puree, oats, protein powder, and a blend of warm spices, offering a fall-inspired treat that's both indulgent and nutritious.

Ingredients:

- 1/2 cup canned pumpkin puree

- 1 cup oats

- 1/4 cup vanilla protein powder

- 1/4 cup almond butter

- 1 teaspoon pumpkin spice

- 1-2 tablespoons honey or maple syrup

Instructions:

1. In a bowl, mix pumpkin puree, oats, protein powder, almond butter, pumpkin spice, and honey or maple syrup until well combined.

2. Roll the mixture into bite-sized balls.

3. Refrigerate for at least 1 hour before serving.

Nutritional Information (approximate):

- Calories: 150

- Protein: 7g

- Carbohydrates: 18g

- Fat: 7g

- Fiber: 3g

Chapter 6: Special Occasions and Celebrations

1. Grilled Lemon Herb Salmon

A succulent salmon fillet marinated in a zesty lemon and herb mixture, grilled to perfection. Serve with a side of roasted vegetables for a flavorful and celebratory dish.

Ingredients:

- 4 salmon fillets

- 2 tablespoons olive oil

- Zest and juice of 1 lemon

- 2 cloves garlic, minced

- 1 teaspoon dried thyme

- Salt and pepper to taste

Instructions:

1. In a bowl, mix olive oil, lemon zest, lemon juice, garlic, thyme, salt, and pepper.

2. Coat salmon fillets with the marinade and let them sit for 15-30 minutes.

3. Grill salmon until it flakes easily with a fork.

Nutritional Information (approximate):

- Calories: 250

- Protein: 30g

- Carbohydrates: 2g

- Fat: 14g

- Fiber: 0g

2. Cauliflower and Broccoli Mash

A low-carb alternative to mashed potatoes, this side dish features cauliflower and broccoli blended to a creamy consistency. Perfect alongside grilled chicken or turkey for a special occasion.

Ingredients:

- 1 head cauliflower, chopped

- 1 head broccoli, chopped

- 2 cloves garlic, minced

- 2 tablespoons Greek yogurt

- Salt and pepper to taste

Instructions:

1. Steam cauliflower and broccoli until tender.

2. Blend steamed vegetables with garlic, Greek yogurt, salt, and pepper until smooth.

Nutritional Information (approximate):

- Calories: 120

- Protein: 8g

- Carbohydrates: 20g

- Fat: 2g

- Fiber: 8g

3. Stuffed Bell Peppers with Quinoa and Ground Turkey

Colorful bell peppers filled with a savory mixture of quinoa, lean ground turkey, tomatoes, and spices.

Baked until tender, these stuffed peppers make a satisfying and festive main course.

Ingredients:

- 4 bell peppers, halved and cleaned

- 1 cup cooked quinoa

- 1/2 lb ground turkey

- 1 cup diced tomatoes

- 1 teaspoon cumin

- Salt and pepper to taste

Instructions:

1. Preheat the oven to 375°F (190°C).

2. In a pan, cook ground turkey until browned. Season with cumin, salt, and pepper.

3. Mix cooked turkey with quinoa and diced tomatoes.

4. Stuff bell peppers with the mixture and bake for 25-30 minutes.

Nutritional Information (approximate):

- Calories: 250

- Protein: 20g

- Carbohydrates: 30g

- Fat: 8g

- Fiber: 6g

4. Caprese Salad Skewers

Elegant skewers featuring cherry tomatoes, fresh mozzarella, and basil leaves drizzled with balsamic glaze. A light and refreshing appetizer for special occasions.

Ingredients:

- Cherry tomatoes

- Fresh mozzarella balls

- Fresh basil leaves

- Balsamic glaze

Instructions:

1. Thread cherry tomatoes, mozzarella balls, and basil leaves onto skewers.

2. Arrange skewers on a platter and drizzle with balsamic glaze before serving.

Nutritional Information (approximate):

- Calories: 120

- Protein: 8g

- Carbohydrates: 5g

- Fat: 8g

- Fiber: 1g

5. Lemon Garlic Herb Grilled Chicken

Juicy chicken breasts marinated in a zesty blend of lemon, garlic, and herbs, then grilled to perfection. Serve with a side of steamed asparagus for a delightful and celebratory meal.

Ingredients:

- 4 chicken breasts

- 3 tablespoons olive oil

- Zest and juice of 1 lemon

- 3 cloves garlic, minced

- 1 teaspoon dried oregano

- Salt and pepper to taste

Instructions:

1. In a bowl, mix olive oil, lemon zest, lemon juice, garlic, oregano, salt, and pepper.

2. Coat chicken breasts with the marinade and let them sit for 30 minutes.

3. Grill chicken until fully cooked.

Nutritional Information (approximate):

- Calories: 200

- Protein: 30g

- Carbohydrates: 2g

- Fat: 8g

- Fiber: 0g

6. Zucchini Noodle Alfredo with Grilled Shrimp

A low-carb twist on a classic Alfredo dish, using zucchini noodles instead of pasta. Topped with grilled shrimp, this meal is both indulgent and bariatric-friendly.

Ingredients:

- 2 medium zucchinis, spiralized

- 8 oz shrimp, peeled and deveined

- 1 tablespoon olive oil

- 1/2 cup unsweetened almond milk

- 1/4 cup grated Parmesan cheese

- 2 cloves garlic, minced

- Salt and pepper to taste

Instructions:

1. In a pan, sauté shrimp with olive oil and garlic until cooked.

2. Add zucchini noodles and cook until just tender.

3. Pour in almond milk and Parmesan cheese, stirring until creamy.

4. Season with salt and pepper.

Nutritional Information (approximate):

- Calories: 250

- Protein: 25g

- Carbohydrates: 8g

- Fat: 12g

- Fiber: 3g

7. Mushroom and Spinach Stuffed Chicken Breast

Chicken breasts filled with a savory mixture of sautéed mushrooms, spinach, and garlic, then baked until golden brown. A sophisticated and satisfying entrée.

Ingredients:

- 4 chicken breasts

- 1 cup mushrooms, chopped

- 1 cup spinach, chopped

- 2 cloves garlic, minced

- 1/4 cup low-fat feta cheese

- Salt and pepper to taste

Instructions:

1. Preheat the oven to 375°F (190°C).

2. In a bowl, mix mushrooms, spinach, garlic, feta, salt, and pepper.

3. Cut a pocket in each chicken breast and stuff with the mixture.

4. Bake until chicken is cooked through.

Nutritional Information (approximate):

- Calories: 220

- Protein: 30g

- Carbohydrates: 5g

- Fat: 8g

- Fiber: 2g

8. Cauliflower Crust Margherita Pizza

A guilt-free pizza option featuring a cauliflower crust topped with fresh tomatoes, mozzarella, and basil. A festive and crowd-pleasing dish for special occasions.

Ingredients:

- 1 cauliflower crust (store-bought or homemade)

- 1/2 cup tomato sauce (no sugar added)

- 1 cup fresh mozzarella, sliced

- Fresh basil leaves

- Olive oil for drizzling

Instructions:

1. Preheat the oven according to cauliflower crust instructions.

2. Spread tomato sauce over the crust and top with mozzarella.

3. Bake until the cheese is melted and bubbly.

4. Garnish with fresh basil and drizzle with olive oil.

Nutritional Information (approximate):

- Calories: 220

- Protein: 15g

- Carbohydrates: 15g

- Fat: 12g

- Fiber: 5g

9. Turkey and Vegetable Kebabs

Skewers of lean turkey chunks, bell peppers, onions, and cherry tomatoes, grilled to perfection. Serve with a side of quinoa for a protein-packed celebratory meal.

Ingredients:

- 1 lb lean turkey chunks

- Bell peppers, onions, and cherry tomatoes

- Olive oil

- Lemon juice

- Italian seasoning

- Salt and pepper to taste

Instructions:

1. In a bowl, mix turkey chunks with olive oil, lemon juice, Italian seasoning, salt, and pepper.

2. Thread turkey and vegetables onto skewers.

3. Grill until turkey is cooked and vegetables are tender.

Nutritional Information (approximate):

- Calories: 250

- Protein: 30g

- Carbohydrates: 10g

- Fat: 10g

- Fiber: 3g

10. Berries and Cream Parfait

A delightful dessert parfait featuring layers of mixed berries and a light, protein-rich cream made with Greek yogurt. A refreshing and sweet way to conclude a special meal.

Ingredients:

- 1 cup mixed berries (strawberries, blueberries, raspberries)

- 1 cup non-fat Greek yogurt

- 1 tablespoon honey or a sprinkle of granola

Instructions:

1. In a glass or bowl, layer Greek yogurt with mixed berries.

2. Drizzle with honey or sprinkle with granola.

3. Enjoy this high-protein parfait as a delightful dessert.

Nutritional Information (approximate):

- Calories: 180

- Protein: 15g

- Carbohydrates: 30g

- Fat: 0g

- Fiber: 3g

Chapter 7: Tips for Success

Congratulations on embarking on your gastric sleeve journey! As you navigate the exciting path to better health, these practical tips will guide you through a successful and fulfilling experience. Remember, each step is a triumph, and your commitment to a healthier lifestyle is commendable.

1. Consult with Your Healthcare Team Regularly

Stay connected with your healthcare professionals, including your surgeon, dietitian, and support groups. Regular check-ins ensure that you receive personalized advice, monitor your progress, and address any concerns promptly.

2. Prioritize Protein Intake

Protein is crucial for post-surgery recovery and long-term success. Ensure each meal contains lean protein sources such as poultry, fish, tofu, and legumes to support muscle health and keep you feeling satisfied.

3. Hydration is Key

Sip water consistently throughout the day to stay hydrated. Aim for at least 64 ounces of water daily, but individual needs may vary. Avoid drinking with meals to prevent discomfort and prioritize hydrating between meals.

4. Mindful Eating Practices

Savor each bite by chewing thoroughly and eating slowly. Pay attention to your body's signals of hunger and fullness. Stop eating when you feel satisfied, not overly full, to avoid discomfort and promote healthy digestion.

5. Embrace Nutrient-Dense Foods

Make every bite count by choosing nutrient-dense foods rich in vitamins and minerals. Include a variety of colorful vegetables, fruits, whole grains, and lean proteins to meet your nutritional needs and promote overall well-being.

6. Meal Planning and Prepping

Plan your meals in advance and prepare bariatric-friendly options. Having nutritious meals readily available reduces the temptation of less healthy choices and ensures you meet your dietary requirements.

7. Regular Physical Activity

Incorporate regular physical activity into your routine. Start with gentle exercises and gradually increase intensity as advised by your healthcare team. Find activities you enjoy to make staying active a sustainable and enjoyable part of your life.

8. Celebrate Non-Scale Victories

Acknowledge and celebrate achievements beyond the scale. Whether it's increased energy, improved mood, or achieving fitness milestones, non-scale victories are powerful motivators on your journey.

9. Mind-Body Connection

Explore stress-reducing practices like meditation, deep breathing, or yoga to nurture your mental well-being. A strong mind-body connection contributes to a positive outlook and overall health.

10. Be Patient and Persistent

Weight loss and lifestyle changes take time. Be patient with your progress and stay persistent in making healthy choices. Embrace the journey, celebrate small wins, and remember that sustainable change is a gradual process.

Your commitment to a healthier lifestyle is a journey of self-discovery and empowerment. By incorporating these tips into your daily routine, you set yourself up for success on the path to a vibrant and fulfilling life post-gastric sleeve surgery.

Conclusion

As we reach the closing pages of this cookbook, it's more than just a collection of recipes; it's a testament to your commitment to health, vitality, and a life well-lived. The decision to undergo gastric sleeve surgery marks the beginning of a transformative journey, one that goes beyond the physical and delves into the very essence of who you are.

In the moments you spend in the kitchen, preparing these bariatric-friendly meals, remember that each stir of the spoon, every colorful ingredient, and the aroma wafting through the air is a celebration of your dedication to a healthier you. The flavors on your plate are not just nourishment for your body but a reminder of the strength within you.

As you savor these dishes, crafted with care and tailored for your unique needs, reflect on the progress you've made and the resilience you've shown. You are not just changing what's on your plate; you are rewriting your story—one filled with determination, self-love, and the pursuit of a life filled with joy and well-being.

Beyond the kitchen, this journey is about embracing a newfound sense of freedom. Freedom from old habits that no longer serve you, freedom to move with ease, and freedom to fully embrace the possibilities that lie ahead. It's about creating a life that aligns with your truest self, where every choice is a step toward a brighter, healthier future.

Remember, success is not always measured on a scale. It's in the laughter shared around a table with loved ones, the energy you feel after a nourishing meal, and the confidence that grows with every positive choice. You are not just reclaiming your health; you are reclaiming your life.

As you close this cookbook, know that the journey doesn't end here. It's an ongoing narrative, and you are the author. Keep experimenting with flavors, discovering new ingredients, and savoring the moments that make this journey uniquely yours.

May these recipes continue to inspire you, and may each meal be a reminder of the incredible strength within you. Here's to your wellness, your joy, and the vibrant chapters yet to unfold. Cheers to a life well-lived!

With heartfelt warmth,

Jerry V. Hatcher

About the author

Jerry V. Hatcher is a culinary virtuoso and the creative mind behind a collection of exquisite cookbooks that transcend the ordinary. With a passion for gastronomy and a flair for culinary artistry, Jerry has crafted a series of cookbooks that take readers on a delectable journey through the world of flavors.

Through his cookbooks, Jerry V. Hatcher combines the finest ingredients with meticulous instructions, ensuring every recipe is a delightful masterpiece waiting to be savored. From tantalizing appetizers to mouthwatering main courses and divine desserts, each page is a celebration of culinary excellence.

With a keen eye for detail, Jerry's cookbooks go beyond the recipes, providing valuable tips, techniques, and personal insights that elevate the cooking experience to new heights. Whether you're a seasoned chef or a culinary enthusiast exploring the kitchen for the first time, Jerry's books cater to all skill levels, fostering confidence and creativity in every home cook.

Each recipe in Jerry V. Hatcher's cookbooks is a reflection of his commitment to authenticity and a passion for diverse cuisines. Drawing inspiration from global flavors and local delicacies, Jerry's culinary creations celebrate the richness of cultures and the joy of sharing food with loved ones. Indulge your passion for cooking and elevate your culinary skills with the culinary masterpieces crafted by Jerry V. Hatcher. Get ready to embark on a gastronomic adventure that will leave you hungry for more, one delicious recipe at a time.

My Little Request

If you have gotten to this point, chances are high you have finished this book.

Thank You for Reading My Book!

I love hearing what you have to say.

I need your input to make the next version of this

book and my future books better.

Please take two minutes now to leave a helpful review on Amazon letting me know what you thought of the book

Thank you so much!

- Jerry V. Hatcher